I0774246

The Essential Guide to Mind-Body Calm: 7 Supplements That Will Radically Transform Your Mood

ISBN: 979-8-3220-1419-5

Release Date: 04/05/2024

This book is intended to provide educational information on the subjects discussed. It is not intended to be a substitute for professional medical advice, diagnosis, or treatment. Always seek the advice of your physician or other qualified health provider with any questions you may have regarding a medical condition. The publisher and author are not responsible for any specific health or allergy needs that may require medical supervision and are not liable for any damages or negative consequences from any treatment, action, application, or preparation, to any person reading or following the information in this book.

First Edition

Library of Congress Cataloging-in-Publication Data is available from the Library of Congress.

Printed in the United States of America

Publisher's Cataloging-in-Publication Data

Names: [Adam Gedney, author.

Title: The Essential Guide to Mind-Body Calm: 7 Supplements That Will Radically Transform Your Mood / [Author's Name].

Description: First Edition. | Includes bibliographical references and index.

Subjects: LCSH Supplements. | Mental health. | Stress management. | Mind and body. | BISAC HEALTH & FITNESS / Herbal Medications. | SELF-HELP / Mood Disorders / General.

emotionalsupportsupplements.com

The Essential Guide to Mind-Body Calm

7 Emotional Support Supplements That Will Radically Transform Your Mood

emotionalsupportsupplements.com

Table of Contents

Chapter 1

Understanding Anxiety and the Quest for Calm

First thing, let's get this out of the way – I want to help you feel calm. Actually calm. I know all too well what it feels like to have frazzled nerves from stress, adult responsibilities, relationship conflicts, and the residuals of childhood trauma. We all have our own story of hardship and challenges in life, but there's a common thread between all of us: when we feel stress, from any cause, our bodies enter flight-fight and release cortisol, the stress hormone. There's no

emotionalsupportsupplements.com

escaping, our mind and bodies are deeply connected, and our emotional world affects our bodies, and in return our bodies affect our emotions. This is both the problem and solution. I'll show you how that's true in a little, but for now, what this means then is that there's hope. With a little knowledge we can safely manipulate our bodies to help support our emotional world, support our mental health work, support our ability to be mindful, and to dramatically reduce the amount of anxiety, nervousness, and jitters we feel. Whether it's in social situations, in relationships, at work, or in our day-to-day private life, we all feel the burden of stress –and this takes a toll on our bodies. I know, I've been there. I was enslaved to my cortisol, just like you –until I found the "magic pill". I learned about calming supplements, then dove deep when I learned first-hand that they <u>actually</u> work. Yes, you can actually **feel** the effect certain emotional support supplements have on your nerves. There's no going back for me. Supplementing for calmness has become a crucial part of my quest for calm and emotional intelligence. It's worked for me, and for many others, so I'm confident that with just a little understanding of the most important emotional support supplements you will find what we found. In the pages that follow I'm going to open up a whole new future for you. What's rewarding for me is to share the peace that I've found. If you end up using our emotional support supplements, great, but if not that's ok, I'm just happy you're about to find a little peace.

My name is Adam, and I've dedicated my life to exploring the depths of mental wellness, focusing on the profound impacts of natural emotional support supplements on our neurochemistry and overall health.

In the world we navigate daily, the quest for calm seems more like a distant dream than an attainable reality. For you, I understand that the waves of anxiety and the longing for balance are more than mere concerns; they're a significant part of your life's journey. Together, we'll embark on a journey towards understanding and, most importantly, managing the intricacies of anxiety through a holistic lens.

The Weight of Anxiety

Anxiety isn't just a fleeting feeling; it's a pervasive *experience* that can affect every aspect of your life. Scientific studies have consistently shown the complex interplay between anxiety and our neurochemistry, highlighting how neurotransmitter imbalances can significantly impact our mental state. For instance, a deficiency in GABA, a key neurotransmitter responsible for calming nervous activity, has been linked to increased anxiety levels. Understanding this connection is the first step towards regaining control.

The Mind-Body Connection

The connection between the mind and body is undeniable. Our thoughts and emotions directly influence our physical health, and vice versa. This bidirectional pathway means that by nurturing our bodies with the right nutrients, we can profoundly affect our mental health. Consider the research showing how omega-3 fatty acids can reduce anxiety symptoms by up to 20%, according to a study published in the *Journal of the American College of Nutrition.* This is just a glimpse into the power of emotional support supplements in balancing our mood and improving our overall well-being.

Your Guide to a Calmer Life

As your guide on this journey, I bring not only my expertise but my personal and professional experiences in helping individuals navigate the tumultuous waters of anxiety. Through trial and error, scientific research, and real-life success stories, I've honed in on seven essential emotional support supplements that can support your quest for calm, balance your mood, and reduce anxiety. My goal is not just to present these supplements but to offer a comprehensive understanding of how they interact with your body and mind.

The Path Forward

As we delve into the specifics of each supplement in the coming chapters, remember that the journey to mental wellness is as much about knowledge as it is about *action*. By understanding the neurochemical effects of these emotional support supplements and the

emotionalsupportsupplements.com

importance of the mind-body connection, you'll be equipped to make informed decisions about your health.

It's not just about reducing anxiety; it's about reclaiming your life and finding that elusive calm in the chaos. With each step forward, you'll learn not just to manage anxiety but to thrive in spite of it.

Chapter 2

The Role of Supplements in Mental Health

Having traversed both the scientific realms and the personal experiences of those seeking solace in natural remedies, I invite you to delve deeper into how specific supplements can be instrumental in rebalancing our neurochemistry, thus fostering a serene mind-body connection.

A Scientific Lens on Supplements

The conversation around mental health often circles back to pharmaceuticals, yet the power of natural emotional support supplements remains underexplored. Supplements, rooted in centuries of traditional medicine and now backed by modern science, offer a complementary approach to managing mental health. For instance, a pivotal study published in the *Nutritional Neuroscience Journal* highlighted that magnesium plays a crucial role in reducing anxiety levels by acting on the NMDA receptors, which are crucial for learning and memory. This is a testament to how elemental nutrients can significantly influence our brain's biochemistry. You can see where this is going –if Omega-3s can reduce anxiety by 20%, and omega-3s can reduce it as well, then finding the right supplement can have very significant impacts on your inner world, freeing you from the overwhelm of anxiety.

Bridging the Gap with Neurochemistry

The neurochemistry of anxiety is a complex web of neurotransmitters and hormonal balances. Omega-3 fatty acids have been shown to reduce inflammation and support the production of neurotransmitters like serotonin and dopamine, which are essential for mood regulation. And here's the proof, A landmark study in the *Journal of Clinical Psychiatry* found that participants with higher levels of omega-3s reported feeling less anxious, illustrating the direct link between nutrient intake and mental health.

Mind-Body Synergy

The harmony between our physical and mental states cannot be overstated. The gastrointestinal tract, often referred to as the "second brain," illustrates this connection perfectly. Probiotics, beneficial bacteria found in certain foods and emotional support supplements, can influence our mood and cognitive functions by producing and regulating key neurotransmitters. A review in the *Annals of General Psychiatry* underscores the potential of probiotics in alleviating symptoms of depression and anxiety, paving the way for a gut-brain synergy that promotes overall well-being.

The Journey with Supplements

As we explore the landscape of supplements, it's important to approach with mindfulness and informed consent. While the scientific evidence is compelling, the journey to integrating emotional support supplements into your life should be personalized and should be supervised by a healthcare professional. This ensures not only the efficacy of the supplements but also their harmony with your unique body chemistry.

Your Pathway to Balance

Embarking on this pathway with me, consider the profound impact that even simple adjustments to your supplement intake can have on your mental health. As we move forward, we'll delve into each of the *seven essential emotional support supplements*, examining their roles, benefits, and the science that makes them invaluable allies in our quest for calm.

In this chapter, we've bridged the gap between ancient wisdom and modern science, illustrating the significant role emotional support supplements play in managing anxiety and enhancing mental health. I'm committed to illuminating this path, empowering you with the knowledge and tools to foster a deep, harmonious connection between your mind and body. Next, we'll explore the transformative power of emotional support supplements, step by step, towards a balanced and serene existence.

Chapter 3

Magnesium: The Relaxation Mineral

I'm excited to introduce you to one of nature's most potent antidotes to stress and anxiety: magnesium. Often referred to as the "relaxation mineral," magnesium plays a pivotal role in over 300 biochemical reactions in the body, directly impacting our nervous system and our ability to manage stress. Let's jump into the science, the stories, and the strategies that make magnesium a cornerstone supplement for mental wellness.

The Science of Magnesium and Anxiety

emotionalsupportsupplements.com

Magnesium's role in promoting a calm and balanced mental state is well-documented. It regulates neurotransmitters, which send messages throughout the brain and body, and binds to GABA receptors, promoting calm, reducing anxiety, and facilitating sleep. A landmark study in the *Journal of the American Board of Family Medicine* found that magnesium supplementation could significantly improve symptoms of anxiety and depression, highlighting its potential as a natural and accessible antidepressant option.

Magnesium and the Mind-Body Connection

The link between magnesium and the mind-body connection is profound. By supporting the nervous system and enhancing the quality of sleep, magnesium helps to rejuvenate the body's stress-response system, thereby improving our overall resilience to stress. Furthermore, its role in muscle relaxation is crucial for those who carry physical tension as a result of stress or anxiety, showcasing the interconnectivity between physical and mental health.

Personalizing Your Magnesium Journey

Incorporating magnesium into your wellness routine can be a game-changer. However, it's essential to consider the form of magnesium, as its absorption varies. Magnesium citrate, for example, is known for its bioavailability and efficacy in improving relaxation and sleep. Start with a modest dose, and observe how your body and mind respond, remembering that this journey is deeply personal and should be tailored to your unique needs.

A Note of Caution

While magnesium is generally safe, it's important to consult with a healthcare professional before starting any new supplement regimen, especially if you have existing health conditions or are taking other medications. This ensures that you embark on this path with the best guidance and support, minimizing any risks and maximizing the potential benefits. And fair warning, too much magnesium before you're used to it will likely cause diarrhea. Don't let this stop you though, find the dose that's right for you.

Magnesium: More Than Just a Supplement

emotionalsupportsupplements.com

Embracing magnesium as part of your daily routine is not just about addressing anxiety; it's about nurturing your body's natural ability to find balance and calm. Whether it's through supplementation, diet (think: leafy greens, nuts, and seeds), or lifestyle adjustments that prioritize relaxation, the journey with magnesium is holistic, encompassing all aspects of well-being.

We've explored the remarkable benefits of magnesium, not only as a supplement but as a testament to the power of natural remedies in supporting mental health. I'd like to remind you that every step you take towards incorporating magnesium into your life is a step towards tranquility, balance, and a deeper connection between your mind and body. Let's continue this journey with another powerhouse supplement, moving us toward a calmer, more resilient you.

Chapter 4

Omega-3 Fatty Acids: Brain Health and Beyond

This chapter could change the way you view your diet and its impact on your mental health. We're diving into the world of Omega-3 fatty acids, essential nutrients that play a crucial role in brain health and emotional well-being. Omega-3s are not just another supplement; they are a fundamental component of cellular membranes throughout our body, including those in the brain, influencing everything from mood regulation to cognitive function.

emotionalsupportsupplements.com

Unlocking the Power of Omega-3s

Omega-3 fatty acids, particularly EPA and DHA, are vital for maintaining the fluidity of cell membranes, which is essential for effective cell-to-cell communication. The study in the *Journal of Clinical Psychiatry* highlighted that individuals with higher levels of Omega-3s reported significantly lower levels of anxiety, illustrating the profound impact these fatty acids have on our mental state.

The Neurochemistry of Omega-3s

The relationship between Omega-3s and our neurochemistry is fascinating. These fatty acids help reduce neuroinflammation, a key factor in the development and persistence of anxiety. They also play a role in synthesizing neurotransmitters like dopamine and serotonin, which are critical for mood regulation. This dual action makes Omega-3s a powerful ally in managing anxiety and enhancing overall brain health.

Incorporating Omega-3s into Your Life

Incorporating Omega-3s into your life doesn't just mean taking supplements; it's about holistic dietary changes that include Omega-3-rich foods like fatty fish (salmon, mackerel, sardines), flaxseeds, chia seeds, and walnuts. For those opting for emotional support supplements, aiming for a balance of EPA and DHA is crucial, and as always, consulting with a healthcare professional to tailor the intake to your specific needs is advised.

Beyond the Mind: The Widespread Benefits of Omega-3s

Omega-3s don't just impact our mental health; their benefits extend to heart health, joint health, and beyond. This broad spectrum of benefits underscores the interconnectedness of our body systems and the importance of a holistic approach to health and wellness. It's a vivid reminder that what we feed our bodies can have a transformative effect on our mental and physical well-being.

A Journey Towards Balanced Well-being

emotionalsupportsupplements.com

As we explore the potential of Omega-3 fatty acids together, remember, this journey is about more than just alleviating anxiety. It's about nurturing your body and mind, creating a foundation for lasting health and happiness. With every step, with every choice that brings more Omega-3s into your life, you're taking control of your well-being, moving towards a future where balance, health, and peace of mind are within your reach.

Let's continue to explore and embrace the power of natural emotional support supplements in our journey towards a calmer, more fulfilled life.

Chapter 5

Vitamin D: Sunshine for Your Mood

Let's shine a light on one of the most underrated yet vital nutrients for our mental well-being: Vitamin D. Often celebrated for its role in bone health, this "sunshine vitamin" also plays a crucial role in mood regulation and mental health. Now let's look at the fascinating science and practical steps we need to harness the power of Vitamin D in our journey toward a more balanced, anxiety-free life.

The Science Behind Vitamin D and Mental Health

Vitamin D's impact on our mental health is profound and multifaceted. It's involved in the synthesis of neurotransmitters like serotonin, which affects our mood, sleep, and overall sense of well-being. A study published in the *American Journal of Geriatric Psychiatry* found a significant correlation between low levels of Vitamin D and higher rates of depression and anxiety, highlighting the essential role of Vitamin D in mental health.

Bridging the Mind-Body Connection

Vitamin D receptors are found throughout the brain, including in areas linked to the development of depression and anxiety. This vitamin helps regulate the release of neurotransmitters, which play a key role in mood and cognitive function. Moreover, Vitamin D's anti-inflammatory properties may protect against neuroinflammation, further supporting its role in maintaining mental health.

Optimizing Your Vitamin D Levels

Optimizing your Vitamin D levels goes beyond just supplementing. While supplements can play a crucial role, especially in areas with limited sunlight or during the winter months, incorporating Vitamin D-rich foods into your diet is also essential. Foods like fatty fish, egg yolks, and fortified foods contribute to a balanced diet rich in this vital nutrient.

Moreover, exposing your skin to sunlight for about 10-20 minutes a day can significantly boost your Vitamin D levels, providing the dual benefits of natural light exposure and stimulating the body's Vitamin D synthesis. However, it's important to balance sun exposure with skin cancer risk, emphasizing safe sun practices.

A Note of Caution

While Vitamin D is essential for mental health, it's crucial to find the right balance. Excessive intake of Vitamin D supplements can lead to health issues, including calcium buildup in the blood, which can harm the heart and kidneys. Consulting with a healthcare provider to determine the appropriate dosage based on your current levels and health needs is always advised.

Embracing Vitamin D in Your Journey

Embracing Vitamin D in your journey towards managing anxiety and achieving mental wellness is about more than just taking a supplement; it's about holistic lifestyle changes that invite more "sunshine" into your life, both literally and metaphorically. As we've seen, the benefits of Vitamin D extend far beyond bone health, playing a critical role in our emotional and psychological well-being.

We've looked at the significant role Vitamin D plays in supporting mental health, highlighting its impact on neurochemistry and the mind-body connection. Let's continue to explore the natural pathways to a balanced, anxiety-free life, with Vitamin D as a key component of our journey.

Chapter 6

Probiotics: Gut Health Equals Mental Health

In this chapter, we're delving into the fascinating world of probiotics and their profound impact on mental health. The saying "trust your gut" takes on a whole new meaning as we explore how the health of our gut microbiome can directly influence our mood, stress levels, and overall sense of well-being.

The Gut-Brain Axis: A Two-Way Street

The gut-brain axis represents the complex communication network linking our gastrointestinal tract and brain, a pathway through which the gut and its microbial inhabitants can send and receive signals that influence our emotions and cognitive functions. Scientific research has illuminated this relationship, showing how an imbalance in our gut microbiota can contribute to a range of psychological issues, including anxiety and depression.

One study in the *Gastroenterology* journal found that taking probiotics could reduce anxiety symptoms by influencing the gut-brain axis, showcasing the potential of gut health management as a component of mental health treatment.

Probiotics and Neurochemistry

Probiotics, the beneficial bacteria residing in our gut, play a crucial role in modulating the gut-brain axis. They influence the production and regulation of key neurotransmitters like serotonin and dopamine, which are pivotal for mood regulation. Remarkably, it's estimated that up to 90% of our body's serotonin is produced in the gut, underscoring the gut's potential as a target for mental health interventions.

Incorporating Probiotics into Your Wellness Regimen

Incorporating probiotics into your daily routine can be as simple as adding probiotic-rich foods to your diet—yogurt, kefir, sauerkraut, kimchi, and kombucha are delicious, natural sources. For those with dietary restrictions or preferences, probiotic supplements offer an alternative way to ensure your gut microbiome is well-populated with beneficial bacteria. However, diversity is key—consuming a variety of probiotic strains can provide the broadest benefits, as different bacteria offer different health advantages.

A Balanced Approach to Gut Health

While probiotics are a cornerstone of gut health, they are most effective as part of a holistic approach to wellness that includes a balanced diet rich in fiber, regular exercise, and stress management practices. Remember, the state of our gut microbiome is not just a reflection of our diet but of our overall lifestyle.

Your Gut, Your Ally

emotionalsupportsupplements.com

Obviously the relationship between gut health and mental health is intricate and powerful. By nurturing our gut microbiome with probiotics and mindful lifestyle choices, we're not just improving our digestive health; we're taking significant steps toward reducing anxiety, enhancing our mood, and elevating our overall quality of life.

Let's continue transforming not only how you feel mentally but bolstering your physical health along the way. As we continue to explore the essential emotional support supplements for finding calm, balancing mood, and reducing anxiety, let's remember that sometimes, the key to our well-being lies within us, starting with our gut, and working through our willingness to take action to feel better. You've taken the first step by reading this book. Let's keep going...

emotionalsupportsupplements.com

Chapter 7

Ashwagandha: Ancient Herb for Modern Stress

As we continue our journey through the realm of natural emotional support supplements and their profound impact on mental health, we arrive at a cornerstone of ancient wellness practices: Ashwagandha. Known as a powerful *adaptogen*, Ashwagandha has been used for centuries in Ayurvedic medicine to help the body manage stress and restore balance. I'm Adam, and I'm here to guide you through understanding how this ancient herb can be a beacon of calm in the modern world of stress and anxiety.

The Power of Adaptogens

Adaptogens like Ashwagandha are unique in their ability to help the body resist physical, chemical, and biological stressors. *They work by modulating the production and release of stress hormones from the adrenal glands, enhancing the body's resilience to stress.* This modulation helps maintain homeostasis in the body, potentially reducing the physiological impact of stress and anxiety on our health. Adaptogens are an incredibly important category of emotional support supplements.

Ashwagandha and the Brain

Ashwagandha's effects extend deeply into the neurochemistry of the brain, influencing the regulation of neurotransmitters such as GABA, serotonin, and dopamine, which are crucial for maintaining mood balance. Research, including a study published in the *Journal of Alternative and Complementary Medicine*, has shown that Ashwagandha can significantly reduce levels of stress and anxiety in adults, highlighting its role as a natural *anxiolytic*(drugs used to reduce anxiety).

Incorporating Ashwagandha into Your Routine

Incorporating Ashwagandha into your daily wellness routine can be a game-changer for managing stress and anxiety. Available in various forms, including powders, capsules, and teas, it's essential to start with a low dose to assess your body's response and gradually adjust as needed. Always seek out high-quality, pure Ashwagandha products from reputable sources to ensure the best results.

A Holistic Approach to Stress Management

While Ashwagandha offers remarkable benefits for reducing stress and anxiety, it's most effective when integrated into a holistic approach to wellness. This includes maintaining a balanced diet, engaging in regular physical activity, practicing mindfulness or meditation, and ensuring adequate sleep—all foundational elements that support mental health.

Navigating the Modern World with Ancient Wisdom

This ancient herb offers much-needed support in our fast-paced, often overwhelming modern lives. By embracing Ashwagandha as part of our wellness toolkit, we're not just tapping into the wisdom of ancient practices; we're empowering ourselves to navigate stress with grace and resilience.

In this chapter, we've uncovered the ancient roots and modern benefits of Ashwagandha, highlighting its potential to bring calm and balance to our lives. I encourage you to explore the integration of Ashwagandha into your routine, mindful of the broader spectrum of health and well-being. Let's keep going to discover and apply the powerful principles of natural emotional support supplements in our quest for a calmer, more balanced existence.

Chapter 8

L-Theanine: The Calming Amino Acid

In our exploration of natural emotional support supplements for managing stress, mood, and anxiety, we encounter a remarkable compound that exemplifies the harmony between nature and neuroscience: L-Theanine, my personal favorite. Found primarily in green tea leaves, L-Theanine is an amino acid celebrated for its unique ability to promote relaxation without sedation, making it an invaluable ally in our quest for calm. Let's dive into how L-Theanine can help us navigate the challenges of modern life with a sense of serenity.

The Unique Properties of L-Theanine

L-Theanine stands out for its ability to enhance alpha brain waves, which are associated with a state of relaxed alertness. This effect on brain wave activity helps reduce anxiety and promotes a state of calm focus, invaluable for those moments when you need to de-stress without losing your edge. Research published in the *Journal of Clinical Psychiatry* supports L-Theanine's anxiolytic (anxiety-reducing) effects, showcasing its potential to improve mental health and cognitive function.

L-Theanine and Neurochemistry

Beyond its impact on brain waves, L-Theanine influences neurochemistry by modulating levels of neurotransmitters like GABA, serotonin, and dopamine. These neurotransmitters play crucial roles in mood regulation, anxiety, and overall emotional balance. L-Theanine's ability to increase GABA, in particular, contributes to its calming effects, offering a natural means of anxiety relief without the side effects associated with pharmaceutical GABAergics.

Integrating L-Theanine into Your Wellness Regimen

Incorporating L-Theanine into your daily routine can be as simple as drinking green tea, which offers the added benefits of antioxidants. For those seeking more precise dosages or who prefer not to consume caffeine, L-Theanine emotional support supplements are an effective alternative. Starting with a dose of 100-200 mg per day can provide noticeable benefits, though individual responses vary, and consulting with a healthcare professional is advisable to tailor your approach.

A Balanced Approach to Relaxation

While L-Theanine is a powerful tool for enhancing relaxation and focus, it's most effective when part of a comprehensive wellness strategy. This includes regular exercise, a balanced diet, adequate sleep, and stress management practices like mindfulness or meditation. Yes, I keep stressing that. There's a reason… Together, these elements create a synergistic effect, amplifying the benefits of L-Theanine and supporting overall mental health and well-being.

Embracing Calm in a Chaotic World

L-Theanine offers a gentle yet profound way to enhance relaxation, improve focus, and reduce anxiety, helping us find calm in the chaos of everyday life. I encourage you to explore the benefits of L-Theanine, mindful of the broader context of your wellness practices.

In this exploration of L-Theanine, we've illuminated its role as a natural anxiolytic and its potential to support mental health through neurochemical balance and enhanced brain function. As we continue our journey through the world of natural emotional support supplements, remember that each action step we take is a step toward a more balanced, healthy, and calm life.

emotionalsupportsupplements.com

Chapter 9

B-Complex Vitamins: Essential for Mood and Stress Management

Getting deeper into natural emotional support supplements for enhancing mental wellness, we encounter a group of nutrients pivotal for cognitive health and emotional balance: the B-Complex vitamins. These vitamins play an integral role in almost every aspect of our mental and physical well-being, from energy production to neurotransmitter synthesis. I'm excited to share how these vital nutrients can support your journey towards a calmer, more balanced state of mind.

The Synergy of B-Complex Vitamins

The B-Complex group includes eight essential vitamins: B1 (thiamine), B2 (riboflavin), B3 (niacin), B5 (pantothenic acid), B6 (pyridoxine), B7 (biotin), B9 (folate), and B12 (cobalamin). Each of these vitamins supports the nervous system in unique yet complementary ways, working together to reduce stress, alleviate anxiety, and promote overall mental health. A deficiency in any of these vitamins can lead to increased stress, mood imbalances, and cognitive difficulties.

B-Complex Vitamins and Mental Health

Research highlights the critical role of B-Complex vitamins in mood regulation and stress management. For instance, vitamins B6, B9, and B12 are directly involved in the production and regulation of neurotransmitters such as serotonin, dopamine, and GABA. A study published in *Psychopharmacology* found that supplementation with B-Complex vitamins significantly improved mood and reduced stress in participants within just a few weeks, underscoring the importance of these nutrients in maintaining mental health.

Incorporating B-Complex Vitamins into Your Wellness Routine

Ensuring an adequate intake of B-Complex vitamins can be as straightforward as maintaining a balanced diet rich in whole foods. Leafy greens, fruits, legumes, nuts, seeds, and animal products are all excellent sources of B-Complex vitamins. For those who may have dietary restrictions or increased nutritional needs, B-Complex supplements offer a convenient way to ensure you're meeting your body's demands for these essential nutrients.

A Note of Balance

While B-Complex vitamins are crucial for mental wellness, balance is key. Excessive intake of certain B vitamins, particularly from supplements, can lead to

emotionalsupportsupplements.com

adverse effects. It's important to aim for the recommended daily allowances, adjusting as needed based on your specific health profile and under the guidance of a healthcare professional.

Empowering Your Journey with B-Complex Vitamins

As we've explored, B-Complex vitamins are not just nutrients; they're foundational elements that support our body's stress response, energy production, and neurotransmitter synthesis, all of which are critical for mental health. By prioritizing these vitamins in our diet or through supplementation, we're taking powerful steps towards managing stress, balancing mood, and enhancing our overall sense of well-being.

We just scratched the surface, looking into the critical role of B-Complex vitamins in supporting mental wellness, highlighting how they contribute to a balanced and healthy mind. Consider the importance of these vitamins in your wellness regimen, always striving for balance and mindfulness in your approach to health. Continue to explore the synergy between

emotionalsupportsupplements.com

natural emotional support supplements and lifestyle choices in our journey towards a calmer, more fulfilling life. Here's where to go next...

Chapter 10

Implementing the Plan: How to Integrate These Supplements into Your Daily Routine

As we approach the culmination of our journey together through the world of essential emotional support supplements for finding calm, balancing mood, and reducing anxiety, it's time to focus on practical implementation. Here's how to seamlessly integrate the powerful supplements we've explored into your daily routine, ensuring that you harness their full potential for enhancing your mental wellness.

emotionalsupportsupplements.com

Creating Your Personalized Supplement Plan

The key to successfully integrating emotional support supplements into your life is personalization. Your unique body chemistry, lifestyle, dietary preferences, and specific mental health goals all play a crucial role in determining which supplements are most suitable for you and how they should be incorporated into your daily regimen.

1. **Start with a Foundation**: Begin by assessing your current diet and lifestyle to identify any gaps that emotional support supplements could fill. For instance, if your diet lacks Omega-3-rich foods, considering Omega-3 supplements could be a beneficial starting point.

2. **Prioritize Based on Need**: Focus on the emotional support supplements that address your most pressing concerns. If stress management is your primary goal, starting with Ashwagandha or L-Theanine might be most effective.

3. **Consult a Healthcare Professional**: Before adding any supplements to your routine, consult

with a healthcare provider to ensure they're suitable for you, especially if you're currently taking medications or have underlying health conditions.

Incorporating Supplements into Your Daily Life

Incorporating supplements into your daily life should be convenient and sustainable. Here are some practical tips:

- **Routine**: Tie your supplement intake to daily habits or routines, such as taking them with breakfast or right before bedtime, to ensure consistency.
- **Tracking**: Consider using a journal or an app to track your supplement intake and note any changes in your mood, anxiety levels, or overall well-being. This can help you fine-tune your regimen over time, and you'll be pleasantly surprised when you see just how much these emotional support supplements make a difference.

emotionalsupportsupplements.com

- **Quality Over Quantity**: Invest in high-quality supplements from reputable sources, like those on EmotionalSupportSupplements.com, to ensure you're getting the most benefit from each dose.

Balancing Supplements with Lifestyle Changes

While emotional support supplements can play a crucial role in managing anxiety and balancing mood, I can't emphasize this enough, they are most effective when part of a holistic approach to wellness. It's like 10xing the effects. A holistic approach includes:

- **Diet**: A balanced, nutritious diet can support your mental health from the inside out.
- **Exercise**: Regular physical activity can significantly reduce anxiety and improve mood.
- **Mindfulness and Stress Management Practices**: Techniques such as meditation, yoga, or deep-breathing exercises can enhance the benefits of emotional support supplements by reducing stress and improving mental clarity.

Navigating the Journey Ahead

As you embark on this path of integrating emotional support supplements into your daily routine, remember that the journey to improved mental wellness is ongoing and ever-evolving. Be patient with yourself, and be open to adjusting your plan as your needs and circumstances change.

In this chapter, we've outlined how to thoughtfully and effectively integrate essential supplements into your daily routine, with an emphasis on personalization, quality, and a holistic approach to wellness. This journey is deeply personal and uniquely yours. We've explored powerful tools for enhancing your mental health, but ultimately, the strength lies within you to create a balanced, fulfilling life –taking action is critical.

Chapter 11

Avoiding Pitfalls: Common Mistakes and How to Navigate Them

Embarking on a journey towards improved mental health through natural emotional support supplements is a commendable path, filled with potential and promise. However, like any journey, it's not without its challenges and pitfalls.

Mistake 1: Overlooking the Importance of Diet and Lifestyle

One common mistake is relying solely on emotional support supplements for mental health improvements while neglecting the foundational aspects of diet and lifestyle. WHile you will definitely see results alone, and not insignificant results, emotional support supplements are most effective when used in conjunction with a balanced diet, regular physical activity, and stress-reduction practices, or mental health work.

- **Solution**: View emotional support supplements as part of a holistic approach to wellness. Ensure your diet is rich in whole foods, engage in regular exercise, and practice mindfulness to complement the benefits of supplements.

Mistake 2: Expecting Immediate Results

Another pitfall is expecting immediate or dramatic results from supplement use. While some emotional support supplements can offer quick relief in certain cases(within the first 20 minutes), most work subtly over time to rebalance and support mental health. THis is where journaling can help, as well as mindfulness and awareness of our inner state and inner feelings.

emotionalsupportsupplements.com

- **Solution**: Set realistic expectations and be patient. It can take several weeks or even months to notice significant changes. Consistency is key.

Mistake 3: Not Personalizing Your Supplement Plan

A one-size-fits-all approach rarely works when it comes to emotional support supplements. Each individual's body chemistry, lifestyle, and mental health goals are unique, and what works for one person may not work for another.

- **Solution**: Work with a healthcare professional or therapist to tailor your supplement regimen to your specific needs. Regularly reassess and adjust your plan as necessary.

Mistake 4: Neglecting Quality and Dosage

Not all supplements are created equal. Opting for low-quality supplements or incorrect dosages can diminish their effectiveness and potentially cause harm.

- **Solution**: Invest in high-quality emotional support supplements from reputable sources. Visit EmotionalSupportSupplements.com for our highest quality solutions. Follow recommended dosages and consult with a healthcare provider to determine the optimal amounts for your specific situation.

Mistake 5: Ignoring Potential Interactions

Supplements can interact with medications, other supplements, and even certain foods, leading to decreased effectiveness or adverse effects.

- **Solution**: Always inform your healthcare provider about all supplements and medications you are taking. They can help identify potential interactions and advise on the safest and most effective way to incorporate supplements into your regimen.

Navigating Your Journey with Confidence

While the road to enhancing mental wellness through emotional support supplements can be complex, understanding how to avoid common pitfalls makes the journey smoother and more rewarding. **Remember, the goal is not just to find temporary relief but to build a foundation for lasting mental health and well-being.**

In navigating these challenges, always prioritize balance, patience, and personalization. By doing so, you'll not only enhance the effectiveness of your supplement regimen but also take meaningful strides towards a healthier, more balanced life. EmotionalSupportSupplements.com is here to support you in making informed, thoughtful decisions on your journey to improved mental wellness. Check our articles for in-depth explorations of multiple emotional support supplements, mental health topics, and general health information.

Chapter 12

Success Stories: Real-life Transformations

Embarking on a journey toward better mental health can feel daunting at the outset, but the stories of those who have navigated this path before us offer light and inspiration. In this section let's look at success stories from individuals who have found calm, balance, and reduced anxiety through the thoughtful integration of emotional support supplements into their wellness routines. These narratives not only illustrate the transformative power of natural emotional support supplements but also serve as a testament to the resilience of the human spirit.

emotionalsupportsupplements.com

Anna's Story: Finding Balance with Omega-3s

Anna, a graphic designer in her mid-thirties, struggled with anxiety and mood swings that made her daily life challenging. After researching and consulting with her healthcare provider, she began incorporating high-quality Omega-3 supplements into her regimen. Over the course of several months, Anna noticed a significant improvement in her mood stability and a reduction in anxiety levels, especially during high-stress periods at work. "Omega-3s were a game-changer for me. They helped me find a balance I didn't know was possible," she shares.

Brian's Transformation: Magnesium for Restful Sleep

Brian, a retired veteran, faced long-standing issues with sleep and chronic stress, which exacerbated his anxiety. Learning about the benefits of magnesium for relaxation and sleep, he decided to give it a try. With a consistent intake of magnesium before bedtime, Brian experienced deeper, more restful sleep, which *dramatically* improved his stress resilience and overall quality of life. "Magnesium has helped me in ways I couldn't have imagined. It's like I've been given a new lease on life," Brian reflects.

Cynthia's Journey: Probiotics for Mind and Body

Cynthia, a high school teacher, suffered from digestive issues and anxiety, not realizing the two could be connected. Upon advice from a wellness coach, she added a probiotic supplement to her daily routine. The changes were gradual but profound. Better gut health led to noticeable improvements in her mental clarity and a significant decrease in anxiety. "I never knew my gut had so much power over my mind. Adding probiotics was a simple step that made a big difference," Cynthia explains.

David's Experience: L-Theanine for Focused Calm

David, an entrepreneur, often found himself overwhelmed by the demands of his startup. Struggling to manage stress and maintain focus, he discovered

L-Theanine. This supplement helped him achieve a state of calm focus, enabling him to tackle challenges without the usual anxiety. "L-Theanine has been a critical tool in my stress management toolkit. It helps me stay calm and focused, no matter what comes my way," says David.

Embracing Your Own Success Story

These stories are just a few examples of how integrating natural emotional support supplements, alongside lifestyle changes, can lead to significant improvements in mental health and well-being. Each journey is unique, highlighting the importance of personalization and patience in the pursuit of balance and calm.

As you reflect on these narratives, remember that your own success story is within reach. With informed choices, consistent effort, and a holistic approach to wellness, you too can experience the transformative effects of natural emotional support supplements on your mental health journey. Let these stories inspire

emotionalsupportsupplements.com

you to explore, adapt, and persevere as you navigate your path toward a more balanced, fulfilling life.

Chapter 13

Conclusion: Your Journey to a Calmer, Happier Life

As we reach the conclusion of our journey together, it's important to reflect on the ground we've covered and look ahead to the paths still to be explored. It's been my privilege to serve as your guide through the world of natural emotional support supplements, sharing insights into how they can support your quest for calm, balance, and reduced anxiety. This journey, however, does not end here. It's a continuous process of learning, adapting, and growing toward the best versions of ourselves.

The Power of Natural Supplements

Throughout this journey, we've delved into the science behind natural emotional support supplements and their profound impact on mental health. From the calming effects of Magnesium and L-Theanine to the mood-balancing benefits of Omega-3s and B-Complex vitamins, we've seen how these natural allies can support our neurochemistry and enhance our mind-body connection. Remember, the choice to incorporate emotional support supplements into your wellness routine should be informed, intentional, and reflective of your individual health needs and goals.

The Importance of a Holistic Approach

One of the key lessons we've explored is the importance of a holistic approach to mental wellness. Supplements are a valuable tool in our arsenal, but they are most effective when combined with a healthy lifestyle, including a balanced diet, regular physical

emotionalsupportsupplements.com

activity, adequate sleep, and stress management practices. Embracing this comprehensive approach ensures that you're not just treating symptoms but nurturing your overall well-being.

Personalization and Patience

Every individual's journey to mental wellness is unique. What works for one person may not work for another, underscoring the importance of personalization in your wellness plan. Be patient with yourself as you navigate this journey. Change often comes gradually, and setbacks are part of the process. Stay committed, be flexible in your approach, and remember that progress, no matter how small, is still progress.

Looking Forward

As you move forward, armed with knowledge and insights about natural emotional support supplements and their role in achieving mental balance, remember that your journey to wellness is ever-evolving. Continue to educate yourself, consult with healthcare

emotionalsupportsupplements.com

professionals, and listen to your body. Your path to a calmer, happier life is paved with the choices you make each day to support your mental and physical health.

A Final Word of Encouragement

My hope for you, as we conclude our time together in this book, is that you feel empowered, informed, and inspired to take control of your mental health through natural means. The journey may be challenging, but it is also incredibly rewarding. Remember, you're not alone in this journey. The steps you take today toward integrating natural emotional support supplements into your life are steps toward a brighter, more balanced future.

Thank you for allowing me to be a part of your journey to a calmer, happier life. May the road ahead be filled with peace, balance, and well-being!

Adam - *Certified Professional Coach*

emotionalsupportsupplements.com